Acknowledgement

I am incredibly appreciative of everyone who helped make "Menopause Reset: Embracing Change, Empowering Life" possible. Their assistance, inspiration, and knowledge have been vital all along the way.

I want to start by sincerely thanking my family, friends, and loved ones for their continuous support and compassion. Your support for me and our endeavor has served as a constant source of inspiration.

Thank you to the committed staff at the publishing company for their arduous work in making this book a reality. This process has been made significantly more enriching by your professionalism and enthusiasm for knowledge dissemination.

I would like to express my gratitude to the specialists and professionals who kindly provided their knowledge and insights on menopause in order to enhance the content of this book. Your knowledge has given the information you've provided more substance and authority.

Thank you for your trust, readers, and women starting their own menopause journeys. My honest wish is that "Menopause Reset" will be a supportive and empowering companion during this period of life change.

Last but not least, I want to thank all the women who have opened up and shared their personal menopause stories and experiences. Your candor and sincerity have served as a beacon, showing us all the inner strength we each possess.

This book was a collective effort, and I am grateful for everyone's encouragement and input in making it what it is today. May "Menopause Reset" inspire women to embrace change and live strong lives both during and after menopause.

I sincerely appreciate you all,

Esther Campbell

Abstract

The comprehensive manual "Menopause Reset" equips women with the knowledge and resources they need to successfully manage the menopausal transition. It addresses the relational, emotional, and physical elements of this momentous life shift using a holistic approach. The book provides useful advice on how to deal with menopausal symptoms, practice self-care, retain intimacy, and cultivate deep connections at this time. "Menopause Reset" shines a beacon of knowledge and support for women going through menopause, pointing them in the direction of a balanced and empowered life by promoting open communication, self-compassion, and a positive outlook. It offers insightful information and professional guidance to help readers through this changing stage with assurance and empowerment. It is a must-read for any woman approaching or going through menopause, as well as for their spouses and loved ones.

Table of contents

Chapter 1

INTRODUCTION

Welcome to "Menopause Reset: Embracing Change, Empowering Life," a transformative guide designed to help you navigate the wonderful journey of menopause with grace and resilience. Menopause signifies the end of one chapter and the beginning of another. It's a natural and empowering time of life, although it can also come with its own obstacles and uncertainties. In this book, we will cover the physical, emotional, and relational components of menopause, giving you practical ways to manage symptoms, prioritize self-care, and develop meaningful connections with loved ones.

Embrace the power of communication as we delve into preserving closeness and navigating emotional upheavals throughout this transforming time. Together, we will explore the significance of self-care and fostering your entire well-being, encouraging you to embrace change and personal growth.

Join us as we celebrate the strength and wisdom of women who have handled menopause with resilience and tap into professional ideas to guide you on your own inspiring path.

Empowerment is at the heart of "Menopause Reset," and our objective is to equip you with knowledge, compassion, and a positive outlook as you embrace this new chapter of your life. Get ready to start a joyful and powerful life during and beyond menopause. It's time to embrace the great lady you are and embrace all that lies ahead. Let's begin this transformative journey together!

Chapter 2

Understanding the Menopausal Transition

The menopausal transition, commonly known as menopause, is a normal biological process that signals the end of a woman's reproductive years. It is a major era of a woman's life that typically happens in her late 40s or early 50s, but the exact time might vary for each individual. This transition is marked by a reduction in the synthesis of reproductive hormones, mainly estrogen and progesterone, leading to different physical and emotional changes.

1. Perimenopause: The menopausal transition generally begins with perimenopause, which can persist for several years before menopause itself.

During perimenopause, hormone levels fluctuate, and women may experience irregular menstruation periods along with numerous symptoms such as hot flashes, night sweats, mood swings, and changes in libido.

2. Menopause: Menopause is formally diagnosed when a woman has not had a monthly cycle for 12 consecutive months. At this moment, the ovaries cease to release eggs, and estrogen and progesterone production drastically diminish. Menopause is a natural aspect of aging, and it signifies the end of a woman's capacity to conceive naturally.

3. Postmenopause: The phase after menopause is referred to as postmenopause. During this time, menopausal symptoms like hot flashes and mood

swings may begin to lessen, but certain consequences of hormonal shifts can continue. It is crucial for women to continue emphasizing their health and well-being during postmenopause.

4. Common Symptoms: The menopausal transition can bring about a range of symptoms, including hot flashes, night sweats, vaginal dryness, changes in sleep patterns, mood swings, irritability, exhaustion, and memory lapses. These symptoms can vary in intensity and length for each woman.

5. Impact on Bone Health: Estrogen plays a critical role in preserving bone density. During menopause, the fall in estrogen levels might raise the risk of osteoporosis, a disorder characterized by brittle and weak bones. Women are recommended to make

efforts to promote their bone health through a balanced diet and frequent exercise.

6. Emotional Well-being: Menopause can also influence a woman's emotional well-being due to hormonal variations and the response to substantial life changes. Emotional support and self-care techniques can be valuable during this era.

7. Therapy alternatives: For women having severe or disruptive menopausal symptoms, numerous therapy alternatives are available. Hormone replacement therapy (HRT) can help reduce symptoms by adding estrogen and/or progesterone. However, the decision to take HRT should be made after speaking with a healthcare physician, as it may involve certain dangers and considerations.

Understanding the menopausal transition is vital for women to navigate this significant life shift with understanding and empowerment. By being aware of the physical and mental changes that follow menopause, women can take proactive actions to manage symptoms, prioritize their health, and embrace this new chapter in their lives.

Chapter 3

Hormonal Changes and Their Impact on the Body

Hormonal changes are a feature of the menopausal transition and can dramatically damage a woman's body in many ways. The key hormones involved in menopause are estrogen and progesterone, which play crucial functions in the female reproductive system and overall health. As women age and enter menopause, the levels of these hormones vary and fall, leading to many physical and emotional changes.

Estrogen: Estrogen is a vital female sex hormone involved in regulating the menstrual cycle, supporting bone health, and keeping good skin and hair. During menopause, the ovaries generate less estrogen, leading to irregular menstruation cycles and finally ending completely.

Progesterone: Progesterone works in concert with estrogen to control the menstrual cycle and prepare the uterus for pregnancy. During menopause, progesterone production also drops, adding to menstrual abnormalities.

Menstrual alterations: As hormone levels fluctuate, women may experience alterations in their menstrual cycles during perimenopause. Periods may become irregular, with changes in flow and duration, until eventually ending altogether in menopause.

Vasomotor Symptoms: Hormonal variations can induce vasomotor symptoms, such as hot flashes and night sweats. These unexpected feelings of heat can cause perspiration and discomfort, influencing sleep quality and everyday activities for some women.

Vaginal Changes: Decreased estrogen levels can lead to vaginal dryness and thinning of the vaginal walls, causing discomfort during sexual intercourse and raising the risk of vaginal infections.

Bone Health: Estrogen plays a critical role in preserving bone density. As estrogen levels fall, women become more prone to bone loss, increasing the risk of osteoporosis, a disorder characterized by brittle and weak bones.

Skin and Hair: Estrogen contributes to skin flexibility and moisture retention, as well as hair thickness and health. Reduced estrogen levels after menopause can lead to dry skin, wrinkles, and thinning hair.

Mood and Emotions: Hormonal changes can influence mood and emotions, leading to mood swings, impatience, and anxiety throughout menopause. Fluctuating hormone levels can alter neurotransmitters in the brain, contributing to these emotional swings.

Cognitive Function: Estrogen is believed to have a protective influence on cognitive function. Some women may experience memory lapses or difficulties concentrating during menopause due to hormonal imbalances.

Understanding the impact of hormonal changes on the body is vital for women going through menopause. While these changes are a natural part of aging, they can be tough to manage for some women. Seeking support from healthcare practitioners, maintaining a healthy lifestyle, and researching treatment choices can help ease symptoms and promote overall well-being during this transitional phase of life.

Chapter 4

Menopause Symptoms

The menopausal transition, spanning perimenopause, menopause, and postmenopause, is a phase of life that brings about numerous physical and emotional changes due to hormonal shifts. Recognizing the symptoms linked to each stage will help women better understand and handle this crucial life transition.

Perimenopause Symptoms: Irregular menstruation Cycles: One of the defining indicators of perimenopause is variation in menstruation patterns, such as shorter or longer cycles, heavier or lighter flow, or missing periods.Hot Flashes and Night Sweats: Vasomotor symptoms, such as hot flashes and night sweats, are frequent during perimenopause, creating sudden feelings of heat and perspiration.Mood Swings: Hormonal variations can lead to mood swings, impatience, and anxiety during this phase.Changes in Libido: Some women may report a decrease or volatility in their sexual drive.Vaginal Changes: Vaginal dryness and pain during intercourse may occur due to decreased estrogen levels.Sleep Disturbances: Perimenopausal women may have trouble getting or staying asleep, leading to interrupted sleep patterns.Menopause Symptoms: Absence of Menstruation: Menopause is formally diagnosed if a woman has not had a menstrual cycle for 12 consecutive months.Hot Flashes and Night Sweats: These vasomotor symptoms may linger into menopause for some women.Vaginal Dryness: Reduced estrogen levels can lead to chronic vaginal dryness and discomfort.Sleep Issues: Sleep difficulties may remain throughout menopause, compromising general well-being and daily functioning.Emotional Changes: Mood swings and irritation might continue following menopause due to hormonal alterations.Postmenopause Symptoms:Stabilization of Menopause Symptoms: As hormone levels stabilize, some symptoms, including hot flashes and night sweats, may diminish in intensity or frequency.Vaginal Changes: Vaginal dryness and discomfort may continue, although they can be controlled with suitable therapy.Bone Health Concerns: Postmenopausal women should be cautious about preserving bone health to prevent osteoporosis.Emotional Well-being: While mood swings may reduce, some women may endure emotional alterations as they adapt to the changes in this postmenopausal phase.It is vital to remember that each woman's menopausal experience is unique, and the severity and length of symptoms might vary. If women have disruptive or worrying symptoms during the menopausal transition, receiving help from a healthcare expert is vital. Treatment alternatives, lifestyle improvements, and support can be adjusted to fit individual requirements and facilitate a smoother journey through perimenopause, menopause, and postmenopause.

Chapter 5

Navigating Hot Flashes and Night Sweats: Coping Strategies and Remedies

Hot flashes and night sweats are common vasomotor symptoms revealed by many women throughout the menopausal transition. These rapid episodes of heat and perspiration can be uncomfortable and disruptive to daily life and sleep. Here are some coping tactics and cures to help handle hot flashes and night sweats:

Dress in Layers: Wearing lightweight, breathable clothing in layers enables quick modifications when a heat flash arises. Natural textiles like cotton can help absorb sweat and keep you comfy.

Stay Cool: Keep your living and sleeping areas cool by employing fans or air conditioning. Keeping a cold pack or a moist cloth available to apply to your neck or forehead during a hot flash might also bring relief.

Manage Stress: Stress can provoke hot flashes for some women. Practicing relaxation techniques such as deep breathing, meditation, yoga, or tai chi can help reduce stress and the frequency of hot flashes.

Avoid inducing Foods and Beverages: Spicy foods, caffeine, alcohol, and hot beverages might induce hot flashes in some people. Identifying and avoiding such triggers might help control symptoms.

Stay Hydrated: Although it may seem paradoxical, staying hydrated can help regulate body temperature and minimize the intensity of hot flashes.

Regular Exercise: Engaging in regular physical activity has been demonstrated to help reduce the frequency and intensity of hot flashes. Choose exercises that you enjoy and are appropriate for your fitness level.

Hormone Replacement Therapy (HRT): For some women, hormone replacement therapy can effectively manage hot flashes and nocturnal sweats. HRT involves the use of estrogen or a combination of estrogen and progestin. It is vital to examine the risks and benefits with a healthcare physician before adopting HRT.

Non-Hormonal Therapies: Some non-hormonal drugs, such as some antidepressants or blood pressure medications, have been proven to help relieve hot flashes. Consult with a healthcare provider to explore relevant solutions.

Herbal Remedies: Some herbal supplements, like black cohosh and evening primrose oil, have been used to control menopausal symptoms, including hot flashes. However, their efficacy can vary across individuals, so consult with a healthcare provider before utilizing them.

Acupuncture: Some women get relief from hot flashes through acupuncture sessions. This ancient Chinese medicine procedure includes putting small needles into certain places on the body.

Keep a Symptom Diary: Tracking your hot flashes and night sweats in a diary can help uncover patterns and causes, enabling you to make lifestyle adjustments accordingly.

Remember that treating hot flashes and night sweats may require a combination of methods and solutions.If these symptoms significantly impair your daily life or quality of sleep, talking with a healthcare specialist is vital to exploring appropriate treatment choices and assistance customized to your requirements.

Chapter 6

Managing mood swings and anxiety

Experienced throughout the menopausal transition might be tough to navigate. Hormonal variations, coupled with big life changes, can lead to mood swings and increased anxiety for some women. Here are some tips for controlling mood swings and anxiety during this phase:

Education and Awareness: Understanding that mood swings and anxiety are common symptoms of menopause can help normalize the experience. Being aware of the hormonal changes and their potential impact on emotions can assist in managing these variations.

Seek Support: Talk to friends, relatives, or a support group about your feelings and experiences. Having a support network can provide emotional affirmation and comfort during this period of transformation.

Practice Mindfulness and Relaxation Techniques: Mindfulness meditation, deep breathing techniques, and progressive muscle relaxation can help reduce stress and increase emotional well-being. Engaging in these routines frequently can boost your ability to manage mood swings and anxiety.

Regular Exercise: Physical activity has been demonstrated to have positive impacts on mood and mental well-being. Incorporate regular exercise, such as walking, yoga, or swimming, into your regimen to improve your overall mental health.

Prioritize Self-Care: Taking care of oneself is vital during the menopausal transition. Engage in hobbies that bring you joy and relaxation, whether it's reading, gardening, or spending time with loved ones.

Maintain a Healthy Diet: A balanced diet rich in fruits, vegetables, whole grains, and lean proteins can improve your general well-being. Limiting coffee, alcohol, and sugary meals may also help calm mood swings.

Limit Stressors: Identify sources of stress in your life and focus on finding strategies to decrease or manage them. Setting reasonable expectations and boundaries might help decrease anxiety.

Cognitive Behavioral Therapy (CBT): Consider receiving professional help from a therapist trained in CBT. This sort of treatment can assist in identifying and confronting negative thought patterns that contribute to mood swings and anxiety.

Hormone Replacement Therapy (HRT): For some women, hormone replacement therapy may help stabilize mood swings and decrease anxiety by replenishing hormones. Discuss the potential advantages and hazards of HRT with a healthcare provider.

Consult a Healthcare practitioner: If mood swings and anxiety dramatically impair your everyday life and well-being, don't hesitate to consult a healthcare practitioner. They can examine your symptoms, provide individualized recommendations, and explore relevant treatment alternatives.

Remember that everyone's menopausal experience is unique, and handling emotional shifts may require a variety of tactics. Be patient and compassionate with yourself as you navigate this transitional time, and know that seeking assistance and professional counseling are vital steps in improving mental well-being during menopause.

Chapter 7

The Menopause Diet

As women go through the menopausal transition, dietary choices play a critical role in promoting hormonal balance and overall well-being. Appropriate nutrition can help ease menopausal symptoms, improve bone health, manage weight, and promote mental stability. Here are some crucial components of the menopausal diet:

Phytoestrogen-Rich Foods: Phytoestrogens are plant chemicals that can mimic estrogen in the body and help balance hormone levels.

Calcium and Vitamin D: To maintain bone health and lower the risk of osteoporosis, focus on calcium- and vitamin D-rich meals. Dairy products, leafy greens, almonds, and fortified foods are excellent suppliers of these nutrients.

Omega-3 Fatty Acids: Found in fatty fish (such as salmon, mackerel, and sardines), flaxseeds, chia seeds, and walnuts, omega-3 fatty acids can help reduce inflammation and improve heart health.

Antioxidant-Rich Foods: Incorporate a variety of colorful fruits and vegetables into your diet to benefit from their antioxidant capabilities. Berries, oranges, bell peppers, broccoli, and spinach are wonderful choices.

Healthy Fats: Include sources of healthy fats, such as avocados, olive oil, nuts, and seeds, to support brain function, hormone production, and overall health.

Limit Processed Foods and Sugar: Minimize processed foods and sugary snacks, as they can contribute to weight gain, inflammation, and swings in energy levels.

Stay Hydrated: Drink enough water throughout the day to maintain proper hydration and support bodily functioning.

Reduce Caffeine and Alcohol: Limiting caffeine and alcohol intake can help reduce hot flashes and encourage better sleep.

Monitor Portion Sizes: During menopause, metabolism may slow down, making it vital to be cautious of portion sizes to maintain a healthy weight.

Regular Meals and Snacks: Eat regular, balanced meals and integrate healthy snacks to maintain consistent blood sugar levels and minimize energy collapses.

Avoid Crash Diets: Restrictive diets can be bad for general health and may exacerbate menopausal symptoms.

Listen to Your Body: Pay attention to how your body responds to particular meals and alter your diet accordingly. Every woman is different, so it's crucial to identify what works best for you.

Remember that the menopause diet is not about severe restrictions but rather adopting a balanced and healthy approach to help your body during this transitional era. Consulting with a licensed dietician or healthcare provider can provide individualized recommendations based on your specific needs and health goals. By adopting conscious food choices and prioritizing a nutrient-rich diet, women can enhance their health and well-being during menopause and beyond.

Chapter 8

Exercise and Fitness for Menopause

Engaging in regular physical activity is vital throughout menopause to promote bone density, cardiovascular health, and overall well-being. As women age and go through hormonal changes, exercise can play a crucial role in controlling menopausal symptoms and reducing the risk of certain health issues. Here's how exercise can assist menopausal women:

Maintaining Bone Density: Weight-bearing workouts, such as walking, running, dancing, and resistance training, can help preserve bone density and lower the risk of osteoporosis. These activities promote the bones to become stronger and denser, which is especially crucial after menopause when estrogen levels decline, harming bone health.

Cardiovascular Health: Menopause is associated with an increased risk of heart disease and cardiovascular disorders. Regular cardiovascular exercises like brisk walking, swimming, cycling, and dancing can help improve heart health, reduce blood pressure, and control weight.

Weight Management: Hormonal changes during menopause can lead to weight gain, particularly around the belly. Regular exercise can aid in weight management by burning calories and improving metabolism.

Mood and Emotional Well-Being: Exercise has been found to release endorphins, which can help enhance mood and lessen symptoms of worry and melancholy. Engaging in physical activity can positively improve mental well-being throughout menopause.

Joint Health: Menopause may also bring about joint soreness and stiffness. Low-impact workouts like yoga, Pilates, and swimming can help increase joint flexibility and minimize discomfort.

Sleep Quality: Regular physical exercise might contribute to improving sleep quality, which is typically disrupted during menopause due to hormonal changes and night sweats.

Enhancing muscular Strength: Strength training routines utilizing resistance bands or free weights can help maintain and develop muscular mass. This is significant because muscle mass tends to decline with age and hormonal changes.

Flexibility and Balance: Activities like yoga and tai chi can enhance flexibility, balance, and coordination, which can help reduce the risk of falls and accidents.

Social connection: Joining fitness classes or clubs can provide opportunities for social connection and support, which can be useful for emotional well-being during menopause.

Consult with a Healthcare practitioner: Before starting a new exercise regimen, especially if you have any current health concerns, consult with a healthcare practitioner or a fitness professional to confirm that the chosen activities are safe and appropriate for your individual needs.

Incorporating a combination of cardiovascular activities, weight training, and flexibility exercises into your weekly program can offer the most benefits throughout menopause.

Remember that exercise is not only excellent for physical health but also plays a significant role in supporting mental and emotional well-being throughout menopause.

Chapter 9

Tips for Restful Nights During Menopause

Getting adequate and restful sleep is vital for overall health and well-being, particularly during menopause, when hormonal changes can alter sleep habits. Here are some recommendations to help women prioritize sleep and increase the quality of their rest during this transitional phase:

Create a Relaxing Bedtime Ritual: Establish a peaceful bedtime ritual to communicate to your body that it's time to wind down. Activities like reading, having a warm bath, performing relaxation exercises, or listening to calming music might help you relax and prepare for sleep.

Stick to a Consistent Sleep Schedule: Try to go to bed and wake up at the same time every day, especially on weekends. This helps balance your body's internal clock and increases the quality of your sleep.

Create a Comfortable Sleep Environment: Make sure your bedroom is favorable to sleep. Keep the room cool, dark, and silent. Invest in a comfy mattress and pillows that support your body.

Limit Screen Time Before Bed: The blue light emitted by screens might interfere with your body's generation of melatonin, a hormone that governs sleep. Avoid using electronic devices like cell phones, tablets, and computers at least an hour before bedtime.

Avoid Stimulants: Limit the intake of caffeine and avoid drinking it close to bedtime, as it might disrupt sleep. Similarly, be aware of alcohol intake, as it can also interfere with sleep patterns.

Manage Hot Flashes: Hot flashes and nocturnal sweats can impair sleep. Keep a fan or a cool pack beside your bedside to help ease discomfort during these bouts.

Consider Sleepwear: Choose breathable and moisture-wicking sleepwear to help minimize night sweats and keep you comfortable throughout the night.

Practice Stress Reduction: Menopause can be a stressful time, and stress can influence sleep quality. Engage in relaxation techniques like deep breathing, meditation, or yoga to reduce tension and encourage better sleep.

Stay Active During the Day: Regular physical activity might enhance sleep quality. However, avoid strenuous exercise close to bedtime, as it may make it harder to fall asleep.

Be Mindful of Food and Drink: Avoid heavy meals and excessive fluid intake close to bedtime to prevent discomfort during the night. Some women find that a light snack, such as a tiny piece of fruit or a handful of nuts, can be helpful.

Seek Medical Advice: If you continue to experience sleep problems despite attempting these methods, consider addressing your sleep concerns with a healthcare specialist. They can help uncover any underlying sleep issues and offer specific recommendations.

By prioritizing sleep and adopting healthy sleep habits, women can promote their general well-being and successfully handle the challenges of menopausal sleep problems. It may take time and patience to find what works best for you, but investing in restful nights can substantially benefit your physical and emotional health during this changing season of life.

Chapter 10

Maintaining Bone Health

As women age, bone health becomes a vital part of overall well-being, especially during the menopausal transition when estrogen levels fall. Osteoporosis, a disorder characterized by weak and brittle bones, can increase the risk of fractures and alter mobility. Here are some approaches to help preserve bone health and avoid osteoporosis:

Calcium-Rich Diet: Calcium is vital for creating and maintaining strong bones. Incorporate calcium-rich foods into your diet, such as dairy products (milk, cheese, yogurt), leafy green vegetables (kale, broccoli), fortified plant-based milks, and calcium-enriched meals.

Vitamin D: Vitamin D is needed for calcium absorption and bone health. Spend time outdoors in the sun to naturally produce vitamin D, and consider adding vitamin D-rich foods to your diet, such as fatty fish (salmon, mackerel), fortified meals, and supplements if needed.

Regular Weight-Bearing Exercise: Engage in weight-bearing exercises that put stress on your bones, such as walking, running, dancing, and stair climbing. These activities promote bone growth and assist in maintaining bone density.

Strength Training: Incorporate resistance exercises utilizing free weights, resistance bands, or weight machines. Strength training helps grow and maintain muscle mass, which is vital for maintaining bone health.

Quit Smoking: Smoking is potentially dangerous to bone health, as it can lead to decreased bone density. Quitting smoking can greatly enhance your bones and general health.

Limit Alcohol Intake: Excessive alcohol use might significantly affect bone health. Limit your alcohol intake to develop stronger bones.

Avoid Excessive Soda Consumption: Colas and other carbonated beverages with phosphoric acid can interfere with calcium absorption. Limit consumption to improve bone health.

Bone Density Testing: Discuss bone density testing with your healthcare professional, especially if you have risk factors for osteoporosis.

Assess Fall Risks: Take measures to prevent falls, as fractures can be particularly serious for women with osteoporosis. Ensure a safe living environment, use handrails, and consider balance exercises.

Hormone Replacement Therapy (HRT): For women at higher risk of osteoporosis, hormone replacement therapy (HRT) may be explored. Estrogen therapy can help retain bone density, but it comes with possible hazards. Discuss the advantages and dangers with your healthcare provider.

Calcium and Vitamin D Supplements: If you struggle to get enough calcium and vitamin D through your diet, supplements can be a beneficial complement to maintain bone health. Consult with your healthcare provider to establish the right dosage.

Remember that bone health is a lifelong responsibility. By implementing these techniques, women can retain strong bones and lower the risk of osteoporosis and fractures as they age. It's crucial to work in conjunction with healthcare experts to analyze individual risk factors and design a specific plan to promote bone health during the menopausal and postmenopausal years.

Chapter 11

Understanding Cardiovascular Risks

Menopause might have significant effects on heart health, as hormonal changes during this transitional phase may affect the cardiovascular system. Estrogen serves a protective role in the heart, and its loss during menopause may increase the risk of certain heart-related disorders. Here are some things you need to know about menopause and heart health:

Cardiovascular Risks: Women are generally at a lower risk of heart disease compared to men until menopause. However, following menopause, the risk of heart disease grows dramatically, and the risk becomes comparable to that of men.

Estrogen's Role: Estrogen has a favorable impact on the cardiovascular system. It helps maintain healthy blood vessel function, lowers cholesterol levels, and enhances blood flow. When estrogen levels diminish during menopause, these protective effects decrease.

Atherosclerosis: Atherosclerosis is the buildup of plaque in the arteries, narrowing them and reducing blood flow. Estrogen helps prevent atherosclerosis; however, after menopause, the chance of plaque development increases.

Hypertension: During menopause, blood pressure may rise due to hormonal changes, weight gain, and decreasing estrogen levels.

Cholesterol Imbalance: Menopause can lead to adverse changes in cholesterol levels, including a drop in HDL (good cholesterol) and an increase in LDL (bad cholesterol) and triglycerides, contributing to heart disease risk.

Metabolic Syndrome: Menopause can be associated with metabolic syndrome, a cluster of disorders that includes abdominal obesity, high blood pressure, insulin resistance, and poor lipid profiles.

Vasomotor Symptoms: Hot flashes and night sweats can alter sleep quality, leading to sleep deprivation, which may impact heart health.

Smoking: Menopausal women who smoke are at higher risk for heart-related problems.

Family History: A family history of heart disease can enhance a woman's heart disease risk during menopause.

Lifestyle Factors: Adopting a heart-healthy lifestyle is vital during menopause to lower cardiovascular risks. This involves regular exercise, maintaining a healthy weight, eating a balanced diet, controlling stress, and not smoking.

Regular Health Checkups: Menopausal women should schedule regular health checkups, including blood pressure, cholesterol, and blood sugar screenings, to monitor their heart health.

Hormone Replacement Therapy (HRT): Hormone replacement therapy (HRT) may be administered to control menopausal symptoms and perhaps aid with specific cardiovascular risks. However, the decision to use HRT should be based on an individual assessment of its advantages and dangers.

Understanding the cardiovascular risks linked with menopause is vital for women to take proactive steps to maintain heart health. By adopting a heart-healthy lifestyle, getting regular medical checkups, and remaining updated about the latest research and therapies, women can lessen the impact of menopause on heart health and enhance their overall well-being throughout this life transition.

Chapter 12

Hormone Replacement Therapy (HRT)

Hormone Replacement Therapy (HRT) involves the use of medications that contain hormones, typically estrogen and/or progesterone, to supplement the declining hormone levels during menopause. HRT is used to manage menopausal symptoms and may have potential benefits and risks. Here are the pros, cons, and types of hormone replacement therapy:

Pros of Hormone Replacement Therapy:

Symptom Relief: HRT can effectively alleviate menopausal symptoms such as hot flashes, night sweats, vaginal dryness, and mood swings, improving the quality of life for many women.

Bone Health:HRT can help prevent bone loss and reduce the risk of osteoporosis in some women.

Cardiovascular Benefits: In some cases, HRT may have cardiovascular benefits, including improved cholesterol levels and reduced risk of heart disease.

Vaginal Health: HRT can improve vaginal health by reducing dryness and discomfort, making sexual activity more comfortable for some women.

Cons of Hormone Replacement Therapy:

Increased Breast Cancer Risk: Long-term use of combined HRT (estrogen and progestin) has been associated with a slightly increased risk of breast cancer. However, the overall increase in risk is small and depends on factors such as the duration of HRT use and individual risk factors.

Blood Clot Risk: HRT, particularly oral estrogen, may increase the risk of blood clots, including deep vein thrombosis (DVT) and pulmonary embolism (PE).

Stroke Risk: Some studies have suggested a slightly increased risk of stroke in women using HRT, particularly in older age groups.

Gallbladder Issues: HRT may increase the risk of gallbladder disease, particularly in women who already have underlying risk factors.

Types of Hormone Replacement Therapy:

Estrogen Therapy (ET): This type of HRT involves using estrogen alone for women who have undergone a hysterectomy (removal of the uterus). Estrogen therapy is available in various forms, including pills, patches, creams, gels, and sprays.

Estrogen-Progestin Therapy (EPT): EPT is recommended for women who still have their uterus. It combines estrogen and progestin to protect the uterine lining from the effects of estrogen, which can increase the risk of uterine cancer. EPT is available in various forms, including pills, patches, and creams.

Bioidentical Hormone Therapy: Bioidentical hormones are chemically identical to the hormones naturally produced in the body. They are available in customized forms prepared by compounding pharmacies. While some women prefer bioidentical hormones, their safety and effectiveness have not been extensively studied.

Low-Dose HRT: Doctors may prescribe the lowest effective dose of hormones to manage menopausal symptoms and reduce potential risks.

Before considering HRT, it is essential for women to have a thorough discussion with their healthcare provider. The decision to use HRT should be based on individual factors, including menopausal symptoms, health history, age, and personal preferences. For many women, HRT can provide relief from bothersome menopausal symptoms and improve overall well-being, but it should be used cautiously and for the shortest duration possible. Regular follow-up with a healthcare provider is crucial for monitoring the benefits and risks of HRT over time.

Chapter 13

Herbal Supplements and Natural Remedies for Menopause

For women seeking alternatives to hormone replacement therapy (HRT) during menopause, several herbal supplements and natural remedies are available. These options aim to alleviate menopausal symptoms and support overall well-being. It's essential to consult with a healthcare provider before using any herbal supplements to ensure safety and efficacy, especially if you have pre-existing health conditions or are taking other medications. Here are some non-hormonal alternatives for menopause:

Black Cohosh: Black cohosh is one of the most well-known herbal supplements for menopause. It is believed to have mild estrogen-like effects and may help alleviate hot flashes, night sweats, and mood swings in some women.

Soy Isoflavones: Soy isoflavones are compounds found in soy products that have mild estrogen-like effects. Some studies suggest that soy isoflavones may help reduce hot flashes and support bone health.

Red Clover: Red clover contains compounds called phytoestrogens, which may have estrogen-like effects in the body. Red clover supplements have been studied for their potential to reduce menopausal symptoms.

Dong Quai: Dong quai is a traditional Chinese herb often used to support women's health during menopause. It is believed to have mild estrogen-like effects and may help with hot flashes and menstrual irregularities.

Evening Primrose Oil: Evening primrose oil contains gamma-linolenic acid, which may help with skin dryness and support overall skin health during menopause.

Chasteberry (Vitex): Chasteberry is an herb that may help regulate hormonal imbalances and alleviate symptoms such as breast tenderness and mood swings.

Maca Root: Maca root is an adaptogenic herb that may help improve energy levels, mood, and libido during menopause.

St. John's Wort: St. John's Wort is a natural antidepressant that some women find helpful for managing mood swings and mild depression during menopause.

Mind-Body Techniques: Mindfulness meditation, yoga, and relaxation exercises can help reduce stress and improve overall well-being during menopause.

Lifestyle Changes: Adopting a healthy lifestyle, including regular exercise, a balanced diet, and adequate sleep, can positively impact menopausal symptoms and overall health.

It's important to note that herbal supplements are not regulated in the same way as prescription medications, and their quality and potency may vary among different brands. Some herbal supplements can interact with medications or have contraindications for certain medical conditions, so always consult with a healthcare provider before adding them to your regimen.

While herbal supplements and natural remedies may offer relief for some women, their effectiveness can vary. What works for one individual may not work for another. Therefore, finding the right combination of non-hormonal alternatives often involves a process of trial and error. Working with a knowledgeable healthcare provider can help you make informed decisions and tailor a holistic approach to manage menopausal symptoms effectively.

Chapter14

Boosting Memory and Mental Clarity during Menopause

During menopause, hormonal fluctuations can impact cognitive function, leading to changes in memory, concentration, and mental clarity for some women. While these changes are typically mild and temporary, there are several strategies to support brain health and boost memory and mental clarity during this transitional phase:

Regular Exercise: Engaging in regular physical activity has been shown to benefit brain health. Exercise increases blood flow to the brain, promotes the release of neuroprotective chemicals, and enhances cognitive function.

Mindful Eating: A balanced diet rich in antioxidants, omega-3 fatty acids, and nutrients can support brain health. Foods such as fatty fish, nuts, seeds, berries, leafy greens, and whole grains are excellent choices.

Cognitive Stimulation: Engage in mentally stimulating activities, such as puzzles, brain games, reading, learning a new skill, or taking up a musical instrument. These activities challenge the brain and help maintain cognitive function.

Quality Sleep: Ensure you get enough restful sleep every night, as sleep is crucial for memory consolidation and overall brain health.

Stress Management: Practice stress-reduction techniques like meditation, deep breathing exercises, or yoga to promote mental clarity.

Social Engagement: Stay socially active and maintain strong connections with friends and family. Social interactions can enhance cognitive function and emotional well-being.

Brain-Training Apps: Utilize brain-training apps and online programs specifically designed to enhance memory, attention, and cognitive skills.

Limit Alcohol and Smoking: Excessive alcohol consumption and smoking can impair cognitive function. Limiting or avoiding these substances can benefit brain health.

Multitasking: Minimize multitasking, as it can lead to reduced focus and memory retention. Instead, prioritize tasks and focus on one thing at a time.

Seek Professional Support: If cognitive changes significantly impact daily life, consider seeking the advice of a healthcare provider or a neurologist to rule out any underlying conditions and receive appropriate guidance.

Remember that menopause-related cognitive changes are a natural part of the aging process and are often temporary. While these strategies can help support brain health and cognitive function, it's essential to approach them with patience and consistency. Embracing a holistic approach to overall well-being, including physical activity, a balanced diet, mental stimulation, and stress reduction, can contribute to maintaining memory and mental clarity during menopause and beyond.

During menopause, hormonal fluctuations can lead to various changes in the skin and hair. Here are some essential tips for burnishing your body's changes during this phase:

Hydration: Drinking plenty of water and using moisturizers with ingredients like hyaluronic acid can help maintain skin hydration.

Sun protection: The skin becomes more susceptible to sun damage due to hormonal changes. Always wear sunscreen with broad-spectrum protection, even on cloudy days, to prevent premature aging and reduce the risk of skin cancer.

Gentle cleansing: Use mild, non-drying cleansers to avoid stripping the skin of natural oils.

Anti-aging ingredients: Look for skincare products with retinoids or peptides to support collagen production and reduce fine lines and wrinkles.

Hair care: Menopause can lead to hair thinning and loss. Consider using volumizing hair products and avoiding excessive heat styling.

Nutritious diet: A balanced diet rich in vitamins, minerals, and antioxidants can benefit both the skin and hair. Foods like fruits, vegetables, and omega-3 fatty acids can support skin health.

Stress management: Practice relaxation techniques like yoga, meditation, or deep breathing to reduce stress levels.

Exercise: Regular physical activity improves blood circulation, which can benefit skin health. It also helps maintain a healthy weight, which can positively impact hormonal balance.

Hormone replacement therapy (HRT): Some women opt for HRT to manage menopausal symptoms, which can also have positive effects on the skin and hair. Consult with a healthcare professional to discuss the potential benefits and risks.

Regular check-ups: Visit a dermatologist and discuss any skin concerns you may have during menopause. They can provide personalized recommendations and address specific skin issues.

Remember that menopause is a natural phase, and with proper care and self-compassion, you can embrace and support your body's changes effectively.

Chapter 15

Intimacy and Sexuality: Addressing challenges and finding pleasure

Maintaining intimacy and sexuality is an essential part of a woman's general well-being during this transitional time of life. Menopause can bring about different physical and emotional changes that could affect a woman's sexual desire and experience. Addressing these obstacles and obtaining enjoyment can be achieved through numerous strategies:

Communication with Partner: Openly fighting the changes and challenges experienced throughout menopause with your partner is vital. Sharing your feelings and concerns will promote understanding and support, offering a safe space to explore intimacy together.

Education and Information: Educate yourself and your partner about menopause and its potential implications for sexuality. Understanding the physical and emotional changes can lessen anxiety and provide insight into strategies to negotiate intimacy more effectively.

Seek expert Guidance: Consider consulting a healthcare expert, such as a gynecologist or a sex therapist, who specializes in menopause and sexuality. They can offer specialized guidance and solutions to solve unique difficulties.

Hormone Therapy: Some women may find relief from menopausal symptoms, including reduced libido, through hormone therapy. Discuss this option with a healthcare provider to discover if it's good for your unique needs.

Lubrication and Moisturizers: Vaginal dryness is a typical concern during menopause, reducing sexual comfort and enjoyment. Using water-based lubricants or vaginal moisturizers can help enhance intimacy and lessen discomfort.

Mind-Body Techniques: Engage in relaxation techniques like mindfulness, yoga, or meditation to manage stress and increase general well-being. Reducing stress can favorably improve sexual desire and enjoyment.

Pelvic Floor Exercises: Strengthening the pelvic floor muscles through exercises like Kegels can enhance sexual experience and boost orgasmic response.

Experimentation and Sensuality: Embrace a spirit of exploration and sensuality in the bedroom. Try new things, explain your desires, and be open to experimenting with different forms of closeness that offer pleasure and joy.

Self-Care and Positive Body Image: Practicing self-care and creating a positive body image can boost confidence and enhance the sensation of pleasure and closeness with yourself and your partner.

Patience and Understanding: Be patient with yourself and your partner as you negotiate these changes. Remember that closeness and sexuality can grow over time, and it's necessary to adjust to the new sensations and problems with compassion and understanding.

By embracing a proactive and open attitude toward sustaining intimacy and sexuality, women during menopause can continue to experience meaningful and gratifying intimate relationships with themselves and their partners. The remedy relies on communication, seeking professional support, and being attentive to the changes that come with this transitional life stage.

Chapter 16

Menopause and relationships: Communicating with partners and love ones

Menopause can significantly impact relationships, and effective communication with partners and loved ones is crucial during this phase. Here's a guide to navigate this transitional period together:

Educate Your Partner: Start by educating your partner about menopause and its potential effects on physical and emotional well-being. Help them understand that menopause is a natural phase of life and may bring about changes in mood, energy levels, and sexual desire.

Open and Honest Communication: Share your experiences and feelings openly with your partner. Be honest about any challenges you may be facing, such as hot flashes, mood swings, or changes in libido.

Empathy and Support: Encourage your partner to express their feelings and concerns about menopause's impact on the relationship. Show empathy and offer support as you both navigate this new territory together.

Patience and Flexibility: Menopause can be a rollercoaster of emotions and physical changes. Be patient with each other and understand that adapting to these changes may take time. Be flexible in finding new ways to connect and show affection.

Seek Emotional and Practical Support: Lean on each other for emotional support, and remember that it's okay to ask for help when needed. Be willing to support each other practically, such as by sharing household responsibilities or seeking assistance with childcare.

Be Mindful of Triggers: Menopause can sometimes amplify emotions, leading to disagreements. Be mindful of potential triggers and try to approach conflicts with empathy and understanding.

Maintain Intimacy: Keep the lines of communication open regarding intimacy and sexual needs. Discuss any changes or challenges honestly, and explore ways to maintain intimacy and pleasure together.

Seek Professional Help: If communication difficulties persist or become overwhelming, consider seeking the guidance of a relationship counselor or therapist. They can provide valuable tools and strategies to navigate these changes effectively.

Continue Bonding Activities: Engage in activities that bring you both joy and strengthen your emotional connection. Whether it's going for walks, sharing hobbies, or spending quality time together, these bonding activities can help maintain closeness.

Prioritize Self-Care: Encourage each other to prioritize self-care during this time. Taking care of your physical and emotional well-being individually will benefit both partners and the relationship as a whole.

Remember that menopause affects both partners in a relationship, and working together with open communication, empathy, and support is key to maintaining a strong and loving bond during this transformative phase of life.

Chapter 17

Managing stress and embracing self-care

Managing stress and embracing self-care during menopause are crucial for navigating this significant life transition with grace and well-being. Menopause can bring about various physical and emotional changes, and adopting effective strategies for stress management and self-care can greatly improve the overall experience. Here are some tailored strategies for achieving balance during menopause:

Educate Yourself: Learn about menopause and the potential symptoms you may experience. Understanding what's happening in your body can help you cope better with the changes.

Prioritize Sleep: Menopause can disrupt sleep patterns. Create a calming bedtime routine and aim for 7-9 hours of quality sleep each night to support your physical and emotional health.

Balanced Nutrition: Focus on a balanced diet rich in whole foods, fruits, vegetables, and sources of calcium and vitamin D to support bone health and overall well-being.

Stay Hydrated: Drink plenty of water throughout the day to stay hydrated and help manage hot flashes.

Regular Exercise: Engage in regular physical activity, such as walking, yoga, or swimming, to boost your mood, reduce stress, and support bone density.

Mindfulness and Meditation: Practice mindfulness and meditation to manage stress and increase self-awareness. These practices can help you stay present and cultivate a sense of calm.

Hormone Therapy and Treatment Options: If menopausal symptoms are severe, consult with a healthcare professional about hormone therapy or other treatment options that may be suitable for your situation.

Seek Support: Talk to friends, family, or support groups about your experiences. Sharing your feelings and concerns can provide comfort and understanding.

Set Boundaries: Learn to say no and set boundaries to manage your energy and avoid unnecessary stress.

Enjoy Pleasurable Activities: Engage in activities that bring you joy and relaxation, whether it's reading, gardening, or spending time with loved ones.

Laugh and Have fun. Laughter is a natural stress reliever. Spend time with people who make you laugh and enjoy humor in your life.

Practice Breathing Exercises: Deep breathing exercises can help reduce anxiety and promote relaxation during stressful moments.

Embrace Self-Compassion: Embrace self-compassion as you navigate through this transformative phase of life.

Pamper Yourself: Take time for self-care rituals, such as massages, baths, or skincare routines, to nurture your physical and emotional well-being.

Seek Professional Support: If menopausal symptoms are significantly affecting your daily life, consider seeking professional support from a menopause specialist or counselor.

Remember that menopause is a unique journey for each woman, and finding a balanced approach to managing stress and embracing self-care is essential. Be patient with yourself, listen to your body, and prioritize your well-being to navigate menopause with resilience and positivity.

Chapter 18

Empowering yourself through menopause: Embracing this life transition

Empowering yourself through menopause involves embracing this life transition as an opportunity for growth, self-discovery, and personal empowerment. Menopause marks the end of one phase of life and the beginning of another, and it's essential to approach it with a positive mindset. Here are some ways to empower yourself during menopause:

Educate Yourself: Knowledge is empowering. Take the time to learn about menopause, its symptoms, and the changes it brings to your body. Understanding what to expect can alleviate anxiety and empower you to make informed decisions about your health.

Shift Your Mindset: Embrace menopause as a natural and normal part of life. View it as a time of renewal and a chance to focus on self-care and personal growth.

Prioritize Self-Care: Make self-care a priority during this phase of life. Listen to your body's needs and engage in activities that nurture your physical, emotional, and mental well-being.

Communicate Your Needs: Be open and honest with your loved ones about your experiences during menopause. Communicate your needs and seek support when necessary. Sharing your journey can strengthen relationships and create a sense of understanding.

Embrace Change: Menopause may bring physical and emotional changes, but these changes can also be opportunities for personal growth and transformation. Embrace the changes and view them as a chance to redefine yourself.

Set Boundaries: As you navigate menopause, set boundaries to protect your well-being and manage your energy effectively. Learn to say no to things that drain you and prioritize activities that bring you joy and fulfillment.

Seek Support: Sharing experiences and supporting each other can be empowering and validating.

Celebrate Your Achievements: Take time to celebrate your achievements and milestones, both big and small. Recognize your strengths and the wisdom gained from your life experiences.

Practice Self-Compassion: Be gentle and kind to yourself during this phase. Acknowledge that menopause can be challenging, and it's okay to have difficult days. Practice self-compassion and give yourself grace as you navigate this transition.

Explore New Opportunities: Embrace menopause as a time of new beginnings. Explore new hobbies, interests, or career opportunities that you may not have had time for before.

Advocate for Your Health: Be proactive about your health during menopause. Advocate for yourself in medical settings and seek the care and treatments that align with your needs and preferences.

Stay Active and Engaged: Continue to stay active physically and mentally. Engaging in regular exercise and pursuing intellectual interests can boost your confidence and overall well-being.

Remember, menopause is a natural part of the aging process and doesn't define you. Embracing this life transition with empowerment and a positive attitude can lead to a more fulfilling and joyful journey. You have the strength within you to navigate menopause with grace and resilience. Embrace this new chapter of your life with open arms and a sense of empowerment.

Conclusion

Finally, "Menopause Reset" is a strong and inspirational title that compassionately and expertly explores the transforming path of menopause. The physical, emotional, and interpersonal components of this momentous life shift are addressed in this book, which is an invaluable resource.

The book "Menopause Reset" provides readers with useful advice on how to deal with menopausal symptoms, improve wellbeing, and cultivate enduring connections at this pivotal time. The book provides a holistic approach to educating women to embrace menopause with grace and resilience, covering everything from navigating hormonal changes to embracing self-care and preserving intimacy.

"Menopause Reset" reassures its readers that menopause is not a stage to be feared but rather a chance for growth, self-discovery, and personal empowerment. It does this by promoting open communication, self-compassion, and a positive outlook. Women are given the tools and insights in this book to take back control of their health and happiness and to lead lives of balance, joy, and fresh purpose.

"Menopause Reset" serves as a beacon of awareness and support in a world where menopause is frequently misunderstood or stigmatized. It offers women a road map for navigating this transforming path with self-assurance and empowerment. Any woman nearing or going through menopause, as well as their spouses and loved ones, should read it since it provides a sympathetic and knowledgeable viewpoint on this wonderful life transformation